PHYSIOTHERAPY IN COMMON LOWER EXTREMITY CONDITIONS

PHYSIOTHERAPIST'S APPROACH

NIHAR RANJAN MOHANTY

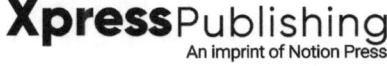

An imprint of Notion Press

XpressPublishing
An imprint of Notion Press

Old No. 38, New No. 6
McNichols Road, Chetpet
Chennai - 600 031

First Published by Notion Press 2020
Copyright © NIHAR RANJAN MOHANTY 2020
All Rights Reserved.

ISBN 978-1-64850-429-7

This book has been published with all efforts taken to make the material error-free after the consent of the author. However, the author and the publisher do not assume and hereby disclaim any liability to any party for any loss, damage, or disruption caused by errors or omissions, whether such errors or omissions result from negligence, accident, or any other cause.

While every effort has been made to avoid any mistake or omission, this publication is being sold on the condition and understanding that neither the author nor the publishers or printers would be liable in any manner to any person by reason of any mistake or omission in this publication or for any action taken or omitted to be taken or advice rendered or accepted on the basis of this work. For any defect in printing or binding the publishers will be liable only to replace the defective copy by another copy of this work then available.

DEDICATED TO

MY BELOVED PARENTS, MY TEACHERS AND MY FRIENDS

Nihar Ranjan Mohanty

BPT; [Swami Vivekanad National Institute of Rehabilitation Training and Research, Cuttack, Odisha, India]

MPT (Sports); [Guru Nanak Dev University, Amritsar, Punjab, India]

Contents

Preface vii

Acknowledgements ix

1. Piriformis Syndrome 1
2. Sciatica 8
3. Patella Tendinopathy 12
4. Myositis Ossificans 19
5. Anatomical Angles 24
6. Common Dislocations Of Lower Limb 29
7. Snapping Joints 37
8. Total Hip Replacement 40
9. Total Knee Replacement 52
10. Special Tests Of Lower Extremity 56

References 69

Preface

This book is a simplified form to describe various approaches and therapeutic interventions of lower extremity common problems via physical therapy. This book is divided into ten chapters. Students and researchers of physical therapy can get the information related to common problems of lower extremity and management principles by physical therapy ready hand from this book. The language is lucid and written in a very concise manner. Point-wise presentation of the subject matters is the strength of this book.

Acknowledgements

First and foremost I would like to thank the almighty for his support and blessings in this long journey.

I would like to express my deepest sense of gratitude to my respected teacher & guide, **Prof. (Dr.) Shyamal Koley**, Head, Department of Physiotherapy, Guru Nanak Dev University, Amritsar, whose knowledge, guidance, and constant encouragement and deep insight without which this book would not have found its final shape.

I would like to thank my **Mother**, for all her support, guidance, motivation and unconditional love, without which I would have never made it through my book. Along with her my greatest regards goes to my **Father, my sisters and my brothers** for the confidence they had in me and I am at loss of words to convey my appreciation and warm regards to them.

My sincere thanks go to my friends **Avinash Tiwari and Diksha** for helping me in my book and being with me in need.

Nihar Ranjan Mohanty

CHAPTER ONE

PIRIFORMIS SYNDROME

Introduction

- Initially described in 1928, Piriformis Syndrome is essentially compression of the proximal sciatic nerve resulting in neuritis and pain.
- Piriformis syndrome is a condition in which the piriformis muscle becomes tight or spasms, and irritates the sciatic nerve.
- In the majority of humans the piriformis originates at the anterolateral portion of the sacrum and inserts at the proximal femur.
- The sciatic nerve crosses under the piriformis at its origin.

Signs and Symptoms

- Patients with PS typically complain of unilateral gluteal pain radiating down the leg. The patient may have paraesthesias in the distribution of the sciatic nerve and its branches. Typically pain is worse with walking and running. It may also be difficult for the patient to precisely locate the pain.
- Most often described by runners.
- PS has been described occurring after periods of prolonged sitting- many cases have occurred after a patient has undergone upright neurosurgery.
- Causes pain in the buttocks region and may even result in referred pain in the lower back and thigh. Patients often complain of pain deep within the hip and buttocks, and for this reason, piriformis syndrome has also been referred to as "Deep Buttock" syndrome.

Physical Examination

- Most commonly, on physical exam the patient with PS will have pain with deep palpation of the affected gluteal muscle. A straight leg raise, similar to that performed with sciatica, may be positive.

Beaty's Maneuver

- Patient is placed on her nonaffected side.
- The affected leg is bent at the knee and abducted against resistance. This may reproduce the patients pain. Beaty originally developed this maneuver after noticing that PS sufferers often complained of pain with rolling over in bed.
- Pain is also elicited with hip flexion, adduction and internal rotation.
- No one clinical test is completely specific, although all of these are sensitive.

What Causes Piriformis Syndrome?

- Piriformis syndrome is predominantly caused by a shortening or tightening of the piriformis muscle.
- Many things can be attributed to this, they can all be categorized into two main groups.

- Overload (or training errors)
- Biomechanical Inefficiencies

Overload(or training errors)

- Piriformis syndrome is commonly associated with sports that require a lot of running, change of direction or weight bearing activity. However, piriformis syndrome is not only found in athletes. In fact, a large proportion of reported cases occur in people who lead a sedentary lifestyle. Other overload causes include:

1. Exercising on uneven ground;
2. Exercising on hard surfaces, like concrete;
3. Beginning an exercise program after a long lay-off period;
4. Increasing exercise intensity or duration too quickly;
5. Exercising in worn out or ill fitting shoes; and

6. Sitting for long periods of time.

Biomechanical Inefficiencies

- The major biomechanical inefficiencies contributing to piriformis syndrome are faulty foot and body mechanics, gait disturbances and poor posture or sitting habits. Other causes can include spinal problems like herniated discs and spinal stenosis. Other biomechanical causes include:

1. Poor running or walking mechanics;
2. Tight, stiff muscles in the lower back, hips and buttocks;
3. Running or walking with your toes pointed out.

Women are 6 times more likely to get PS- Although more women carry a diagnosis of PS then men; there is as yet, no great research as to why.

Could it be that because of the greater Q angle, women place slightly more stretch on the piriformis- leading to a greater rate of inflammation?

Women often complain of dyspareunia with PS. If the Q angle theory is correct the aggravation of PS would be due to the abduction and external rotation of the hip joints during coitus.

Isn't this just Sciatica?

- Yes! Sciatica is a catch- all term used to describe any pain syndrome with symptoms in the distribution of the sciatic nerve.
- It is important to differentiate sciatica from PS because treatment differs!
- When MDs hear sciatica they think herniated disc- guess where the patient goes then? MRI- and it is likely some pathology will be found, and then the patient is destined for surgery.

MRI, Spine X-Ray and CT

- Anatomical variants can be seen on MRI
- CT can show inflammation
- X-Ray used to rule out spine pathology
- Nerve conduction studies are also frequently performed to assess the sciatic nerve conduction.

Botox

- Botox injection is the latest trend in PS treament.
- A recent study showed that pain significantly improved over baseline in 29 patients receiving low dose botox injection under CT guidance. However, controls were removed from the study when their pain did not improve at the first follow-up. Since most PS will improve over time, this study was essentially uncontrolled, and it is difficult to make conclusions about botox efficacy.
- A second study of 9 women with PS showed that fluroscopically guided botox was more effective in reducing pain than saline immediately after injection.
- The bottom line= the jury is still out whether expensive botox is better at pain relief than good old steroids.

Piriformis Syndrome Prevention

- Prevention is the key when it comes to piriformis syndrome.
- There are a number of preventative techniques that will help to prevent piriformis syndrome, including modifying equipment or sitting positions, taking extended rests and even learning new routines for repetitive activities. However, there are four preventative measures that I feel are far more important and effective.
- <u>Firstly</u>: A thorough and correct warm up will help to prepare the muscles and tendons for any activity to come. Without a proper warm up the muscles and tendons will be tight and stiff. There will be limited blood flow to the hip area, which will result in a lack of oxygen and nutrients for the muscles. This is a sure-fire recipe for a muscle or tendon injury.
- <u>Secondly</u>: rest and recovery are extremely important; especially for athletes or individuals whose lifestyle involves strenuous physical activity. Be sure to let your muscles rest and recover after heavy physical activity.
- <u>Thirdly</u>: Strengthening and conditioning the muscles of the hips, buttocks and lower back will also help to prevent piriformis syndrome.
- <u>Fourthly</u>: Flexible muscles and tendons are extremely important in the prevention of most strain or sprain injuries. When muscles and tendons are flexible and supple, they are able to move and perform without being over stretched. If however, your muscles and tendons are tight and stiff,

it is quite easy for those muscles and tendons to be pushed beyond their natural range of movement. When this happens, strains, sprains, and pulled muscles occur.

For Best Results:

- Runners and other athletes know that stretching feels good! The runner's stretch (or yoga's "pigeon pose) is the best single therapy for PS.
- It isn't complicated- patients need to stretch, indulge in some massage, use a heating pad and some NSAIDs.
- And don't forget the golden rule of sports injury prevention: If it hurts- don't do it!

Gluteus Stretch

Lying down on your back, bend your right knee, and place your left leg over the right leg, resting the outside of the left ankle slightly above the right knee. Place your right hand around the outside of your right thigh and place the left hand around the inside of your right thigh. Lock the two hands together. Now pull forward towards your chest to achieve a stretch in the left gluteus portion of your buttocks. Do the exact opposite to achieve a stretch of the right gluteus portion of the buttocks. Hold each stretch for a minimum of 30 seconds, any less than 15 seconds and the muscle will not conform to the new increase in length. Do 3 reps, 3-6 times a day. Any pain you feel with this exercise should only be a local stretching sensation to the back of your thigh and buttocks area, without aggravating your condition.

Piriformis Stretch

Lying down on your back, bend your right leg and pull up your right knee towards your opposite chest with your left hand. You should feel the stretch in the Piriformis portion of the right buttocks. Do the exact opposite to achieve a stretch of the left Piriformis portion of the buttocks. Hold each stretch for a minimum of 30 seconds, any less than 15 seconds and the muscle will not conform to the new increase in length. Do 3 reps, 3-6 times a day. Any pain you feel with this exercise should only be a local stretching sensation to the back of your thigh and buttocks area, without aggravating your condition.

TFL Stretch

Start with stretching the TFL portion of the left hip and outside thigh. While standing, hold your left hand securely on a solid surface to support your body as you place your left leg past your right until you reach a maximum stretch. Follow this with tilting your upper back to the right side while simultaneously pushing the left side of the hip. Do the exact opposite to achieve a stretch of the right TFL portion of the hip and outside thigh. Hold each stretch for a minimum of 30 seconds, any less than 15 seconds and the muscle will not conform to the new increase in length. Do 3 reps, 3-6 times a day. Any pain you feel with this exercise should only be a local stretching sensation to the TFL portion of the hip and outside thigh, without aggravating your condition.

Calf Stretch

Start with stretching the right Gastrocnemius portion of the right calf area. While standing, place your right leg in front of you and your left foot directly behind you. Place the toes of your right forefoot up against a door or other flat wall surface, keeping your heel down to the floor. Lean your upper body forward to place a stretch on the back of the calf. Do the exact opposite to achieve a stretch of the left calf area. Hold each stretch for a minimum of 30 seconds. Any less than 15 seconds and the muscle will not conform to the new increase in length. Do 3 reps, 3-6 times a day. Any pain you feel with this exercise should only be a local stretching sensation to the calf area of the leg, without aggravating your condition.

Psoas Stretch

Start with stretching the right Psoas muscle. While standing, place your right leg in front of you and your left foot directly behind you as far as you can comfortably stretch it. Shift your lower body forward, while simultaneously pushing your upper body backwards with your arms. Do the exact opposite to achieve a stretch of the right Psoas portion of your front upper thigh area. Hold each stretch for a minimum of 30 seconds. Any less than 15 seconds and the muscle will not conform to the new increase in length. Do 3 reps, 3-6 times a day. Any pain you feel with this exercise should only be a local stretching sensation to the Psoas area of the upper thigh, without aggravating your condition.

Quadriceps Stretch

Stand on your left leg, one knee touching the other. You can hold a chair or the wall to keep you steady if needed. Grab your right foot, using your right hand, and pull it towards your buttock. Hold the position for 20 to 30 seconds, then repeat, switching from your left leg to your right.

NIHAR RANJAN MOHANTY

CHAPTER TWO

SCIATICA

Introduction

Sciatic nerve is the thickest nerve of the body. It is the terminal branch of the lumbo-sacral plexus.

Root value: Ventral rami of L4, L5, S1, S2, S3. It consists of two parts.

Tibial Part: its root value is ventral division of ventral rami-of L4, L5, S1, S2, S3, segments of spinal cord.

Common peroneal part: Its root value is dorsal divsion of ventral rami of L4, L5, S1, S2 segments of spinal cord.

Course: It arises in the pelivis. Leaves the pelvis by passing through greater sicatic formmen below the piriformis to enter the gluteal region.

In the gluteal region, it lies deep to the gluteus maximus muscle, and crosses superior gemellus, obturator internus, inferior gemellus, quadratus femoris to enter the back of thigh, during its short course, it lies between ischial tuberosity and greater trochanter with a convexity to the lateral side. It gives no branches in te gluteal region.

In the back of thigh, it lies deep to bliceps femoris and superficial to adductor magnus.

Termination: It ends by dividing into its two terminal branches in the back of thigh.

Sciatica(sciatic neuritis) - is a set of symptoms including pain that may be caused by general compression and/or irritation of one of five spinal nerve roots that give rise to each sciiatic nerve, or by compression or irritation of the left or right or both sciatic nerves. The pain is felt in the lower back, buttock, and/or various parts of the leg and foot. In addition to pain, which is sometimes severe, there may be numbness, muscular weakness, pins and needles or tingling and difficulty in moving or controlling the leg. Typically, the symptoms are only felt on one side of the body. Pain can be severe in prolonged exposure to cold weather.

Although sciatica is a relatively common form of low back pain and leg pain, the true meaning of the term is often misunderstood. Sciatica is a set of symptoms rather than a diagnosis for what is irritating the root of the nerve, causing the pain. This point is important, because treatment for sciatica or sciatic symptoms will often be different, depending upon the underlying cause of the symptoms.

CAUSES

Sciatica is generally caused by the compression of lumbar nerves L4 or L5 or sacral nerves S1, S2, or S3, or by compression of the sciatic nerve itself. When sciatica is caused by compression of a dorsal nerve root (radix) it is considered a lumbar radiculopathy (or radiculitis when accompanied with an inflammatory response). This can occur as a result of a spinal disk bulge or spinal disc herniation (a herniated intervertebral disc), or from roughening, enlarging, and/or misalignment (spondylolishesis) of the vertebrae, or as a result of degenerated discs that can reduce the diameter of the lateral foramen through which nerve roots exit the spine. The intervertebral discs consist of an annulus fibrosus which forms a ring surrounding the inner nucleus pulposus. When there is a tear in the annulus fibrosus, the nucleus pulposus (pulp) may extrude through the tear and press against spinal nerves within the spinal cord, cauda equina, or exiting nerve roots, causing inflammation, numbness or excruciating pain. Sciatica due to compression of a nerve root is one of the most common forms of radiculopathy.

Pseudosciatica or non-discogenic sciatica, which causes symptoms similar to spinal nerve root compression, is most often referred pain from damage to facet joints in the lower back and is felt as pain in the lower back and posterior upper legs. Pseudosciatic pain can also be caused by compression of peripheral sections of the nerve, usually from soft tissue tension in the piriformis or related muscles (see piriformis syndrome and see below).

DIAGNOSIS

Sciatica is diagnosed by physical examination, neurological testing and patient history, "the diagnostic value of patient history and physical examination has not been well studied" "if a patient reports the typical radiating pain in one leg combined with a positive result on one or more neurological tests indicating nerve root tension or neurological deficit the diagnosis of sciatica seems justified."

The most applied diagnostic test is the straight leg rising test, or Lasègue's sign, which is considered positive "if pain in the sciatic distribution is reproduced between 30 and 70 degrees passive flexion of the straight leg"

If no improvement in symptoms has occurred in six weeks or *red flags* are present, imaging is appropriate. Imaging may include either CT or MRI. MR neurography has been shown to diagnose 95% of severe sciatica patients, while as few as 15% of sciatica sufferers in the general population are diagnosed with disc-related problems. MR neurography may help diagnose piriformis syndrome which is another cause of sciatica that does not involve disc herniation.

SYMPTOMS

The most common symptom from sciatica is pain. Most people describe a deep, severe pain that starts low on one side of the back and then shoots down the buttock and the leg with certain movements. Sciatica can also cause hip pain.

- The pain is usually worse with both prolonged sitting and standing. Frequently, the pain is made worse by standing from a low sitting position, such as standing up after sitting on a toilet seat.
- In most people, the pain is made worse by sneezing, coughing, laughing, or a hard bowel movement. Bending backward can also make the pain worse.
- You may also notice a weakness in your leg or foot, along with the pain. The weakness may become so bad you can't move your foot.

TREATMENT

When the cause of sciatica is due to a prolapsed or lumbar disc herniation 90% of disc prolapses will be resolved with no intervention. Treatment of the underlying cause of the compression is needed in cases of epidural abscess, epidural tumors, and cauda equina syndrome.

Although medications are commonly prescribed for the treatment of sciatica, the UK's National Health Service reports that "There is no good evidence from clinical trials to guide the use of analgesics to relieve pain and disability", and suggests that recommendations for analgesic use are extrapolated from guidelines on low back pain. Research has shown no significant difference between placebo and NSAIDs, analgesics, or muscle relaxants, while evidence for opioids and compound drugs is lacking.

Research has failed to show a significant difference in outcomes between advice to stay active and recommendations of bed rest. Similarly, physical therapy (exercises) has not been found to be better than bed rest.

Elective surgery is the main option for unilateral sciatica and focuses on removal of the underlying cause by removing disk herniation and eventually part of the disc. In a controlled study, surgical intervention was found to have better results after one year but after four and ten year follow ups no significant differences were found.

A comprehensive systematic review found moderate quality evidence that spinal manipulation is effective for the treatment of acute sciatica, however, only low level evidence was found to support spinal manipulation for the treatment of chronic sciatica.

CHAPTER THREE

PATELLA TENDINOPATHY

Introduction

The patellar tendon is located just below the knee cap (patella) and is approximately two finger-breadths wide. The tendon is where the quadriceps muscles at the front of the thigh converge and attach to the shin bone.

The function of the patellar tendon is to transfer the force of the quadriceps muscles, the contraction of which results in the extension (straightening) of the knee. The quadriceps muscles are involved in most activities during football, including running and kicking the ball.

Physiology of Patellar Tendon

- The greatest amount of stress is put through the patella tendon during jumping and, just as importantly, during landing:
- During jumping, a player develops an explosive spring by forceful contraction of the quadriceps muscles, which straighten the knees. Together with the calf muscles, the quads push the player up into the air. As the player lands, the quads help to control the landing by allowing a small amount of knee bending to take place.
- If this type of activity is practiced too much, the strain on the patella tendon becomes too great and there is microscopic damage to the tissue that makes up the tendon. At first, this damage may be too small to cause the player any problems but, if the player continues to over-do jumping activities, the damage will become progressively worse.

Pathology of Patellar Tendinopathy

- Patella tendinopathy is usually characterized by degeneration of the tendon (tendonosis) as evidenced at surgical biopsy:

- This is a breakdown in the tendon, characterized by small, focal lesions within the tendon without an inflammatory response. The degeneration means that the tendon does not possess its normal tensile strength and is liable to rupture with continued sporting activity.
- Apart from sporting overuse, this condition is also associated with ageing. As we get older, our ability to regenerate damaged tissue decreases and the quality of the tendon deteriorates.

Signs and Symptoms

- Patella tendinopathy usually comes on gradually.
- There is pain in the tendon which is worsened by activity.
- The focal areas of degeneration feel tender to touch.
- Often the tendon feels very stiff first thing in the morning.
- The affected tendon may appear thickened in comparison to the unaffected side.

Management

- Overload is bad for tendons but so is drastic underload (i.e. complete rest, plaster).
- Tendinopathy can be cured in a clinical sense.
- The 'art' of managing tendinopathy is being able to teach the patient to *moderately* load the tendon and increase this load gradually as tendon function improves.
- **Eccentric-only exercise** appears to be more helpful than concentric, isometric or a combination
- Most important form of management is LOAD tendon within pain limits (not REST, not overload)

What can you do if you come across problem?

- Consult sports injury specialist
- Give ice therapy
- Tie knee straps
- Ice can be used for analgesia (never apply ice directly to the skin) .
- Early recognition by a doctor or Physiotherapist helps greatly, because the outcome is better if treatment is initiated early.

- The key to recovering from Patellar Tendinopathy is in trying to elicit a healing response without overloading the tendon. This may require rest from sporting activities for up to three months. This is because the collagen tissue, which the body produces to repair the tissue damage, takes three months to lie down and mature. This process may be assisted by treatments that increase the temperature of the tendon, increasing the metabolic activity and thus the healing process in the tendon.

- **Tendinopathy management has changed- Was previously called "tendin*itis*" – *itis* = inflammation**
- Wastreated with rest & stretching.
- NSAIDs (Nurofen & Voltaren) & cortisone injections *were* generally encouraged.
- Surgery was used for many chronic cases.
- Now most of this management is frowned upon.

Off Season Management

- Short rest period
- Start low loading early and slowly build up
- Avoid NSAIDs and cortisone
- Definitely use eccentric exercises
- Decide on any surgery early in off-season
- Don't have any sudden increases in load

In Season Management

- Goal is to stabilise until end-of-season, when curative management is attempted (i.e. very hard to cure in season).
- Reduce non-critical training loads.
- Only use NSAIDs and cortisone if no other option.
- Eccentric exercises if they don't aggravate the problem.
- Don't play all year with local anaesthetic for tendinopathy.

Eccentric Muscle Work

- Any tendinopathy can be treated with eccentric only exercises.

- Sometimes these are easy to do as a single person (tennis elbow, patellar, Achilles)
- Sometimes assistance is required (adductor, hamstring origin etc.)
- Eccentric muscle work refers to a muscle that is lengthening while contracting - a contraction that occurs during movements such as landing and decelerating. Maximal tension is generated in the muscle during the eccentric contraction and this causes the tendon to adapt and get stronger.

Why do eccentric muscle exercises fail?

- Ongoing overload (i.e. players in season, but also those who overload in off season)
- Pathological changes so severe that reversal is not possible with first line treatment.

    (a) Partial rupture-unrepaired
    (b) Calcific changes
    (c) Neovascularisation

Work on nearby deficits

It has been shown that patients with patella tendinopathy have greater incidence of weakness elsewhere.

E.g. for patella tendon, athlete may need to -

- Strengthen calf muscles
- Stretch hamstrings etc.

Drug Treatment

- NSAIDS/ CORTISONE
- APROTININ
- SCLEROSANTS
- NITRATE PATCHES

NSAIDS

- Patellar Tendinopathy is usually degenerative, and infrequently due to an inflammatory response. Therefore, the use of anti-inflammatory

medication (NSAIDs) is not appropriate.
- The action of the NSAIDs can actually be counter-productive, as these drugs inhibit the action of naturally occurring chemicals that mediate a healing response, thus dulling the body's ability to regenerate the damaged tissue

Cortisone

- Used for decades
- Give short-term pain relief
- Weaken the tendon
- Anti-inflammatory but may not be mechanism of action (symptom relief)
- Relieve impingement
- Associated with tendon rupture
- Usually not indicated in patella tendinopathy

Aprotinin injections

- Used in persistent cases
- Injected around the tendon
- Helps to prevent further tendon degeneration.
- MOA-Aprotinin is a protein which inhibits the enzyme 'metalloprotease' that breaks down protein that makes up tendon tissue. This drug is useful as it has been shown that in tendinopathies there is an imbalance between different types of metalloprotease, and Aprotinin addresses this imbalance.
- Few serious side effects as compared to corticosteroids.
- Can be injected several times.

Administration of Aprotinin

- 3ml + 2ml local anaesthetic (multi-dose vial)
- 3-4 injections over 3-6 weeks
- Superficial peri-tendinous technique
- Rest that day, train/play the next
- Many patients get an itch
- Many have improvement within days

- Some don't improve but no apparent 'bounceback'
- Therefore good adjunct to other treatment

What other injection options are there?

- Prolotherapy – irritant only (e.g. dextrose)
- Deliberate tendon irritation (dry needling, U-S guided needling)
- Autologous blood
- Calcium gluconate
- Sclerosant-this therapy is based on that pain is generated by new blood vessels being generated in the injured tissue,by injecting sclerosant we sclerose these vessels and hence minimise the pain generators

Nitrate Patches

- Quarter of Nitrodur GTN patch 5mg/24 hrs e.g. 1.25mg/24 hrs
- If blood pressure low or normal- headaches likely.
- Symptomatic relief

Shock Wave Therapy

- Extracorporeal shock wave therapy (ESWT) has been seen safe and promising
- Used in chronic conditions.
- In conditions where conservative management has failed.
- The athlete will be in supine position with an extended knee and shockwaves will be focused on the painful zone in the tendon or insertion.
- Repetitive application of shockwaves is more effective without than with local anaesthesia

SURGERY

- Used in severe cases of Patella Tendinopathy, which have **failed to respond to six months of supervised rehabilitation with** a physiotherapist, then surgery should be considered. However, this is very much a last resort.

- Surgery involves removing degenerate tendon tissue and trying to restore a tendon to a good level of tensile strength. This means that following surgery the tendon still doesn't have its normal strength and careful rehabilitation is essential.

IMAGING IN TENDINOPATHY

- X-ray shows calcium
- Ultrasound good as dynamic test
- MRI good for Differential diagnosis
- Used to show ruptures
- Don't expect imaging to return to normal
- Many normals have abnormal tendons on US.

Surgery vs. eccentrics for jumper's knee

- Surgery no better than eccentric exercises after 12 months and inferior results prior to this
- Recommend eccentrics over surgery if there is a choice!

REHABILITATION

- Physical therapy including-
- Eccentric quadriceps training
- Water training
- Running on soft ground
- Avoiding jumping on hard surfaces.

PREVENTION

- Training errors should be avoided:
- The intensity, duration and frequency of training should be carefully monitored and gradually progressed, and sudden increases avoided.
- Muscle strength and flexibility should be maintained through regular strengthening and stretching sessions.
- The surface should be appropriate to the sport and it is important to wear the correct footwear.
- Use shoe insoles

CHAPTER FOUR

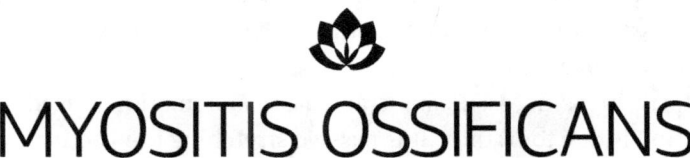

MYOSITIS OSSIFICANS

Introduction

- A very rare progressive disorder involving calcification of muscles, ligaments and tendons.
- It is extra-skeletal ossification. If you have a bad muscle strain or contusion (dead leg!) and it is neglected then you can have Myositis.
- It is usually as a result of impact which causes damage to the sheath that surrounds a bone (periostium) as well as to the muscle.
- Bone will grow within the muscle (called calcification) which is painful. The bone will grow 2 to 4 weeks after the injury and be mature bone within 3 to 6 months.

Incidence

- Most people if not all, have a history of trauma, simple severe blow or series of repeated minor traumas. Condition may be classified according to its location as extra osseous, periosteal or parosteal.
- Haematoma seems to be necessary prerequisite. **Muscles**most often involved are **brachialis, quadriceps femoris and adductor muscles of thigh**.
- Commonly young athletic men are predisposed with Myositis. **Region of elbow is a favorite site**, and when the process appears to restrict elbow motion progressively, ill advised forcible manipulation will cause a widespread involvement.

What causes myositis ossificans?

- Not applying cold therapy and compression immediately after the injury.

- Having intensive physiotherapy or massage too soon after the injury. Use someone who is properly qualified and insured.
- Returning too soon to training after exercise.
- If the ossification is located in the adductor muscles, it is known as **"Prussian's disease"**.
- The term myositis ossificans traumatica is sometimes used when the condition is due to trauma. It is passive stretching then active exercise, is responsible for bone formation.
- The second condition, myositis ossificans progressiva (also referred to as fibrodysplasia ossificans progressiva) is an inherited affliction, autosomal dominant pattern, in which the ossification can occur without injury, and typically grows in a predictable pattern.IP joint of thumb, large toe and spine are liable to fuse. All joint motion is finally lost and patient dies of inter current infection. This condition is very rare.

SYMPTOMS
The list of signs and symptoms mentioned in various sources for Myositisossificans includes:

- Muscle weakness
- Rigid muscles
- Tendon weakness
- Rigid tendons
- Calcium deposits in muscles
- Movement pain
- Tenderness
- Skin swelling over calcified site
- Restricted range of movement
- Pain in the muscle when you use it
- A hard lump in the muscle
- Shortened digits
- Skeletal malformations
- Malformed fingers
- Malformed toes
- Limited joint movement

INVESTIGATIONS

- Radiographs: soft tissue ossification not attached to bone is common.
- X-rays show round mass with distinct peripheral margin of mature ossification & a radiolucent center of immature osteoid & primitive mesenchymal tissue.
- This peripheral maturation, reverse of that seen in a malignant tumor, is characteristic of myositis.
- CT-Scan:
  calcification of the heterotopic ossification proceeds from the outer margin and progresses centrally
- Bone-Scan:
  active myositis appears as intense para-osseous accumulation of tracer activity in acutely damaged muscle on delayed images;
- Prognosis:
  over time, the volume of heterotopic bone will diminish.

TREATMENT

- One of the primary factors that cause a muscle injury to become myositis ossificans is the delay in treatment. This lackadaisical attitude towards treatment increases the chances of developing bone formation. To be precise, ignoring the first line of treatment after a bruise can put a person in the risk zone of calcification. So, taking the treatment as early as possible (in fact immediately) is the safest bet when it comes to substantially minimizing the occurrence of myositis ossificans. Under any circumstances, the treatment must start within two days, once the person has sustained the muscle injury.

Pharmacological

- Treatment of myositis ossificans may include- corticosteroids,
- nonsteroidalanti-inflammatory medications
- narcotic pain medications,
- and surgery
- Anti-inflammatory medications are also effective to treat myositis ossificans, as they relieve the discomfort of the patient. Indomethacin is beneficial as it helps to reduce the pain. Although indomethacin might be available over the counter, taking the consent of the doctor is very important before you start the dosage.

Physiotherapy

***Rest*-** be it hematoma or any other type of physical injury, taking rest as much as possible is always recommended. Keep the injured area immobile for the first 48 hours can not only shorten the recovery time but also inhibit the progression of calcification process inside the muscles. If complete rest is not possible, restricting movements thatput minimal strain onthe area inflicted with damage is recommended. This will insulate the damaged area from excessive pressure, thereby preventing worsening of the injury.

Ice Therapy

In order to treat localized skin inflammation around the injured area use of ice therapy is a good option. As we all know, the inflammation is due to internal bleeding resulting from damage to blood vessels. Application of ice compresses these blood vessels, thereby preventing them from leaking blood. Restricting blood leakage contributes in reducing inflammation of the skin. One can use an ice pack such as a bag of frozen peas and move around the injured site for approximately 15 minutes. You can repeat this session of ice massage 2 - 3 times in a day.

Compression Therapy

Compression therapy too can helpful in managing pain and to speed up healing. The procedure involves wrapping up a soft bandage around the injured site. The patient is bound to experience considerable amount of discomfort when using this compression wrap as it renders support and stability to the damaged muscle.

Elevation

Another effective way to decrease swelling associated with contusion is by keeping the injured site raised well above the heart level. Elevating the damaged limb for a maximum duration of time in the first 72 hours can work wonders to reduce pain and inflammation. Elevation inhibits blood circulation at the injured site and in fact in such a position, the blood is directed away from the damaged area, which encourages healing of pain and inflammation.

Exercise

Certain exercises are recommended to promote flexibility in the injured muscle. Do not attempt exercises immediately after injury. Wait for at least 3 - 4 days after injury and then only begin after consulting with your doctor

- Keep in mind that primary aim of rest, ice therapy, compression and elevation is not only to facilitate recovery but also to prevent muscle injury from advancing to calcification. So, these traditional methods should not be overlooked and treatment should begin without wasting a single minute after the injury.

Surgery

Will surgical removal of abnormal bone formation help to resolve the issue? Not necessarily! Abnormal bone development may begin once again post surgery. To be precise, the bone abnormality may come back to haunt the patient, even after once it has been removed through surgery. Doctors generally wait for 6 to 12 months before considering surgical removal. It is likely to comeback, if it is removed before maturity.

CHAPTER FIVE

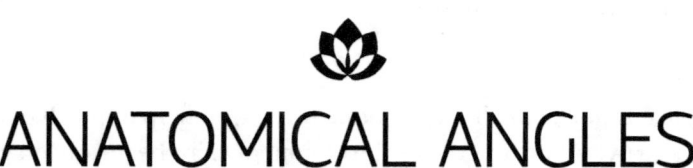

ANATOMICAL ANGLES

Lower Humeral Angle

- It is the Angle between lower articular ends of Humerus to shaft of bone.
- Normal value - 60°.
- Angle disturbed in Diacondylar fracture, Supracondylar fracture, Separation of lower epiphysis.
- *Significances* -- It maintains elbow joint stability, biomechanics of elbow joint and muscle biomechanics of the same.

Carrying Angle

- In extension, the forearm bones make an angle with humerus resulting in an arc which is convex inwards.
- Cause- medial aspect of trochlea extends more distally than lateral aspect result in lateral deviation of ulna.
- *Significance* - In female it is larger as they are having wider pelvis, so , easy arm swing during walking.
- Normal Range- In males, 5° to10°, In females, 10° to 15°.
- It disappears -when forearm pronated and the elbow is in full extension.

   - when supinated forearm flexed against humerus in full elbow flexion.
   Angle disturbed by:
   - Fracture of lower end of humerus.
   - Rupture of the collateral ligaments.

- If the carrying angle increase is called *Cubitus Valgus* and if it is obliterated called *Cubitus Varus*.

In fracture of lateral condyle of Humerus, due to diminished growth of lateral epiphysis results in cubitus valgus deformity. This may result in late *Tardy ulnar nerve palsy*.

- In Supracondylar fracture of Humerus, due to Mal union, distal fragment tilted medially and in internal rotation result in Cubitus Varus called **Gun-Stock deformity with -15° medial**deviation.

Angle of Inclination

It is an angle in frontal plane between an axis through neck and head with longitudinal axis of shaft of femur.

- Normal value – It changes across life span.
- 115° to 135° in adult (Average 120°)
- Pathological increase called Coxa Valga and pathologic decrease called Coxa Vara.
- *Significance* – Normal angle useful for the proper weight transfer from pelvis to lower limb. Abnormal angle increases stress on hip joint and affect posture and gait.

Coxa Valga

- Pathological increase in medial angulation between neck and shaft.
- Causes – Congenital and Hip injury.
- Distance between crest of Ilium and trochanter major is increased.
- Related Posture –

    - Posterior pelvic tilt.
    - Hip in abduction and external rotation.
    - Long ipsilateral leg.
    - Supinated Subtalar joint.

Coxa Vara

- Pathological decrease in medial angulation between neck and shaft of femur.
- Causes – Congenital or Acquired

In Coxa vara the lesion may be:
1) At Epiphysial junction of head and neck. e.g. Slipping of epiphysis
2) In the neck of femur. e.g. Bending- cervical coxa vara.
3) Bending of shaft of femur just below greater trochanter e.g. Rickets Related posture & Deformity -

- Anterior pelvic rotation
- Greater trochanter is raised
- Medial rotation of leg
- Pronated subtalar joint
- Short ipsilateral leg
- Hip Abduction range decrease (B/L scissors gait)

Slipping Of Upper Femoral Epiphysis

Causes- Plane of Epiphysial line is horizontal in childhood but it begins to get more vertical after 10 year.

- The periosteum around the neck of femur becomes thinner during adolescence.
- It exists a pure separation with no fracture of the metaphysis.
- In this type of injury resulting in the deformity suggests a tearing of blood vessels with associated hyperemia.

Torsion Angles of femur

- Angle between an axis through the femoral head and neck with an axis through femoral condyles viewed from top to bottom of femur.
- Normal range – 10° to 20° (adults).
- *Significances* - It maintains hip joint stability, weight bearing biomechanics of hip joint and muscle biomechanics of the same.
- Pathological increase in angle called Anteversion*where*as decrease known as Retroversion.
- *Toeing in* is due to anteverted hip where as *Toeing out* is due to retroverted hip.

Genu Valgum(*Knock – knee***)**

- Medial tibiofemoral angle greater than 185° (Normally 180° to 185°).

- Causes – Rickets, Growth imbalance in femoral condyle, Muscular (Semimembranosus, Semitendinosus) weakness or paralysis, Ligamentous weakness, Secondary to Coxa- vara / flat foot /O.A. knee.
- Lateral aspect presence of Compression forces, whereas medial aspect distraction (tensile) forces.
- It causes excessive pronation of feet as center of gravity during the gait is medial to the subtalar joint.
- Angle depends on the width of pelvis i.e. distance between acetabula.

Genu varum

- Medial tibiofemoral angle is 175° or less.
- Causes – O.A. knee, early weight bearing in children who are fat and heavy.
- It causes increase varus heel strike and greater lateral stress.
- May cause increase stress of lateral knee structures and development of patellofemoral pain.
- Excessive pronation occurs at subtalar joint to allow medial aspect of the foot to make ground contact.
- Lateral aspect presence of distraction (tensile) forces, whereas medial aspect compression forces.

Q - Angle

- The angle between a line connecting ASIS to mid point of patella and extension of line connecting tibial tubercle and midpoint of patella.
- Net effect of pull of Quadriceps can be assessed clinically.
- Normal value – 10° to 15° (with knee full extension). Female> male.
- Any increase in Q angle is thought to increase lateral force on patella.
- With knee flexion it reduces as tibia rotates medially. It also increase when the medial femoral torsion and the lateral tibial torsion are coexist.

Flat Foot

- The arches of foot may be looked upon as angles which are concave downward and convex upward. In Flat Foot, it straightened out.
- *Significances*- Arches help to maintain posture during walking, running and jumping. Also work as shock absorber.

- Causes- Congenital, Traumatic, Muscular and ligament weakness, Drooping of talar head, Pronated foot.

Two types –
1) Congenital or Rigid-Calcaneus found in valgus position, Midtarsal in pronation, Soft tissue contracture with bony changes
2) Acquired or Flexible– Deformity same as first type but it is mobile.

Hallux Valgus

- Abnormal abduction of the first metatarsal with adduction of phalanges.
- Normal first Metatarsophalangeal angle is 8° to 20°.
- Tendon of extensor hallucis longus is shortened and displaced laterally, with mechanical disadvantage, which increases the deformity.

Calcaneal Angle (Bohler's angle)
   Normal Range – 25° to 40°

- A line is drawn from the superior aspect of the anterior to superior aspect of posterior facet. Second line is drawn from the superior aspect of the posterior facet to superior most point of Calcaneal tuberosity.
- *Significance* -Normal obliquity of it is important for weight bearing.

CHAPTER SIX

COMMON DISLOCATIONS OF LOWER LIMB

Hip joint
Stronger joint because of-

- Shape of bones which interlock like ball and socket
- Action of gravity which holds bones together
- Powerful muscles surrounding the joint
- Powerful ligaments stabilizing around
- Smaller activity and ROM

Posterior dislocation
Head of femur is pushed out of acetabulum posteriorly.

- Cause : Car dashboard injury
- Clinical features: History of trauma with flexion, adduction & internal rotation of hip.

  - Marked shortening of leg length
  - Gross restriction of hip movement
  - Head of femur felt as hard mass at gluteal region
  - Associated sciatic nerve palsy

Investigation: X-Ray
Treatment: Closed reduction. Immobilization for 4-8 weeks in – Thomas splint with skin traction, POP hip spica.
Complications:

- Sciatic nerve palsy
- Avascular necrosis femoral head
- Osteoarthritis
- Myositis ossificans

Anterior dislocation
Cause: Legs forcibly abducted & externally rotated, Fall from tree & foot gets stuck and hip abducts excessively.
Clinical features:

- Limb in an attitude of external rotation
- True lengthening with head palpable in groin
- Associated injury to femoral nerve/artery/vein

Treatment: Classical method
Complications: Aseptic necrosis, Post traumatic OA, Neuro vascular injury

Central dislocation
Acetabulum is driven through medial wall of acetabulum towards pelvic cavity.
Cause: Direct blow over trochanter, Epileptic convulsion
Clinical features:

- No limb shortening
- Limb is neutral in position
- Bruising over greater trochanter
- Per rectal examination reveals head of femur

Treatment:

- Reduced by traction with pelvic compression or heavy skeletal traction in 2 directions.
- Traction maintained for 6-8 weeks.
- Physiotherapy

Complications:

- OA
- Recurrence
- Avascular necrosis
- Sciatic nerve palsy
- Superior gluteal artery injury
- Bowel obstruction
- Myositis

Knee Joint
Dislocation of tibia or femur on each other
Cause: Considerable violence, Torn cruciate/collateral ligament.
Patho-anatomy: Strong ligaments hold the joint, if any of them is torn then joint displaces as bony configurations do not provide any strength
Clinical features: Visible deformity, Associated injury to popliteal nerve/artery
Management:

- Open reduction internal fixation with above knee POP for 12 weeks
- Extensive ligament reconstruction
- Physiotherapy

Patella dislocation

1. Congenital dislocation- Patella dislocated at birth

- Associated with abnormality of lateral condyle of femur
- Non reducible dislocation
- Surgical option is not very successful

2. Traumatic or acute dislocation

- Due to direct violence
- Athletic activity – hockey
- Results from sudden contraction of quadriceps with knee flexed or semi flexed.

Clinical features:

- Patella dislocates laterally,
- Inability to straighten the knee,
- Medial condyle of femur is more prominent
- Dislocation may reduce spontaneously but marked tenderness may be present
- Severe pain and swelling

Investigation: X-ray
Management:

- Reduction & immobilization in cylinder cast for 3 weeks
- Surgery
- Physiotherapy

3. Recurrent dislocation

Bone tends to pass outwards, as frequently as knee goes for ROM
Causes:

- Ligament laxity
- Abnormal placed patella
- Small patella
- Genu valgum
- Weak muscles
- Poorly developed lateral femoral condyle

Clinical features: Repeated dislocation, severe pain
Treatment: Hauser's operation: Insertion of patellar tendon is shifted medially & downwards (line of pull of quads shift medially), Patellectomy.

4. Habitual dislocation :

- Patella dislocates every time knee is flexed
- ROM is pain free

Cause:

- Abnormal attachment of iliotibial tract
- Joint laxity syndrome
- Shortened quadriceps
- Neonatal fibrosis of quadriceps due to intramuscular injection

Clinical feature: Abnormal lateral pull on patella on knee flexion
Treatment:

- Extensive lateral releases
- Repair of lax structures medially
- Trans position of tibial tubercle

5. Permanent dislocation :

- Due to untreated childhood / adolescent dislocation
- Patella is permanently dislocated
- Strength of quadriceps is decreased

Treatment:

- Surgery, which aims at à Moving tubercle of tibia with patellar ligament to a more medial position
- Correct knock knee
- Tightening medial patellar ligament
- Increase prominence of lateral femoral condyle
- Physiotherapy

Subtalar dislocation

Dislocation of distal articulations of talus at both talocalcaneal & talonavicular joints

- Lateral dislocation
- Medial Dislocation

Lateral Dislocation

- Calcaneus is displaced lateral to talus
- Talar head lies medially & foot appears pronated

Medial Dislocation

- Foot & calcaneus are displaced medially
- Head of the talus prominent dorsolaterally
- Foot is plantar flexed and is supinated

Investigation: X-Ray
Non Operative treatment:

- Closed reduction is facilitated with knee flexion to relax the gastrocnemius.

Operative Treatment:
Medial dislocations: Open reduction but no need for internal fixation. A short leg cast for 3-4 weeks.
Lateral dislocations: Open reduction. Non weight bearing cast for 3 weeks
Complications:
 - Infection
 - Avascular necrosis

Ankle dislocation
Causes:

- Ligamentous disruption
- Joint hyperlaxity
- Internal malleolar hypoplasia
- Peroneal muscle weakness
- History of prior ankle sprains

4 types of dislocations

- Posterior
- Anterior
- Lateral
- Superior

Posterior (commonest)

- The talus moves in a posterior direction in relation to the distal tibia

- Occurs due to plantar flexion force

Anterior

- Result from the foot being forced anteriorly with the foot fixed

Lateral

- Results from forced rotational forces on the ankle.

Superior

- Force drives the talus upward into the mortice
- Usually due to fall from a height

Physical inspection:

- Significant oedema
- Deformity
- Tenting of the skin by the malleoli
- Tenderness along the joint line

Complications:

- Avascular compromise of the talus
- Permanent sensation or nerve damage
- Tissue necrosis, and gangrene
- Infection
- Myositis
- Late arthritis

Foot (Intertarsal)
Chopart's dislocation
Dislocation of talonavicular & calcaneocuboid joints

Causes: fractures of calcaneus, cuboid & navicular, fall from height, twisting injuries to foot.

Pathoanatomy: foot is dislocated medially & superiorly when it is plantar flexed & inverted lateral displacement during eversion injuries.

Investigation: X-ray
Treatment:

- ORIF to restore & stabilize talonavicular joint
- Open reduction and fusion of calcaneocuboid joint
- Physiotherapy

Tarsometatarsal
Lisfranc's dislocation: one or all metatarsals are displaced from tarsus
Causes: fall from height during horse riding or during windsurfing.
Clinical examination: amount of swelling, location of bruising, areas of tenderness.
Investigations: X-ray (multiple films necessary), CT & MRI scans.
Treatment: casting for 6 weeks, ORIF, Physiotherapy.

CHAPTER SEVEN

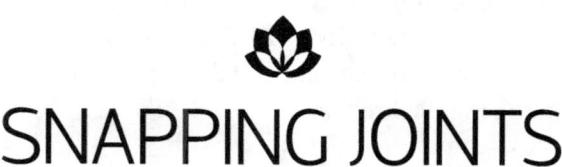

SNAPPING JOINTS

Introduction

- This is a peculiar and rare condition in which a certain movement of a joint is accompanied by an audible click.
- It may occur in a normal joint or more commonly in one the seat of disease.
- In rheumatoid arthritis grating sounds are common in joints; at the knee, for instance creaking are often heard when the joint is flexed and extended.
- We are here only concerned with clicks in healthy joints.

Snapping Hip

- Also known as **coxa saltans, iliopsoas tendinitis or dancer's hip.**
- It is a medical condition characterized by a snapping sensation felt when the hip is flexed and extended.
- This may be accompanied by an audible snapping or popping noise and pain or discomfort.
- Pain often decreases with rest and diminished activity.

Snapping hip syndrome is classified by location of snapping -Internal, external, and intra-articular snapping.
1. Inernal hip snapping:

- It may be caused by slipping of the iliopsoas tendon over the osseous ridge of the lesser trochanter or anterior acetabulum, or the iliofemoral ligament may be riding over the femoral head.

- If due to the iliopsoas tendon or iliofemoral ligament, the snapping often occurs at approximately 45 of flexion when the hip is moving from flexion to extension, especially with the hip abducted and laterally rotated – SNAPPING HIP SIGN or EXTENSION TEST.
- The snap, which may be accompanied by pain or a jerk, is palpated anteriorly in the inguinal region.

2. External hip snapping:

- The snapping may be caused by a tight iliotibial band or gluteus maximus tendon riding over the greater trochanter of the femur.
- This snapping or popping, which tends to be felt more lateral, occurs during hip flexion and extension, especially if the hip is held in medial rotation, and may be made worse if the trochanteric bursa is inflamed.

3. Intra- articular snapping:

- It may be occur when acetabular labral tears or loose bodies, which may be the result of trauma or degeneration.
- In this case, the patient complains of sharp pain into the groin and anterior thigh, especially on pivoting movements.
- Passively, clicking may be felt and heard when the extended hip is adducted and laterally rotated.
- Each of these conditions may be referred to as **SNAPPING HIP SYNDROME.**

Snapping knee

- Recurrent subluxation of mild degree owing to the tibia slipping forward or rotating outwards on the femur in extension. It is common in infants.
- Undue mobility of lateral meniscus.
- Slipping of biceps, semimembranosus, or some other tendon over a bony projection.- usually an exostosis.
- Discoid lateral meniscus.

Slipping peroneus longus

- The tendon of this muscle runs downs to pass behind the external malleolus. It may owe laxity of the peroneal retinaculum slip out of its groove on to the outer surface of the malleolus.
- The condition is painful and may be accompanied by a click.

Trigger finger

- Also known as digital tenosynovaganitis stenosus, this deformity is the result of a thickening of the flexor tendon sheath, which causes sticking of the tendon when the patient attempts to flex the finger.
- A low grade inflammation of the proximal fold of the flexor tendon leads to swelling and constriction in the digital flexor tendon.
- When the patient attempts to flex the finger, the tendon sticks, and the finger "let's go", often with a snap.
- As condition worsens, eventually the finger will flex but not let go, and it will have to be passively extended.
- The condition is more likely to occur in middle aged women, whereas "trigger thumb" is more common in the third or fourth finger.
- It is most often associated with rheumatoid arthritis and tends to be worse in the morning.

Snapping Jaw

- Audible snap in one or other temporo-mandibular joint on opening and closing the mouth.
- It is due to too free movement of the intra articular disc or cartilage.

Snapping Neck

- Occurred where extension of the neck from a flexed position is accompanied by an audible click which is painful and occurs whenever the neck is straightened. It is due to friction between the 5th and 6th cervical spines.

CHAPTER EIGHT

TOTAL HIP REPLACEMENT

Introduction

The hip joint is a type of joint known as a ball and socket joint. The cup side of the joint is known as the acetabulum and the ball side as the head of femur. In a total hip replacement the acetabulum is replaced with a plastic and metal component and the head of the femur is replaced with a metal component which is inserted into the shaft of the femur. Following your operation you will be encouraged to mobilise as soon as possible and you must make sure that you are receiving adequate pain relief to allow you to do this. Normally, you will be sat out of bed the day after the operation with assistance and a walking aid. Unless told otherwise, you should be taking as much weight on your operated leg as you can tolerate.

- Mobility will be progressed during your admission with the physiotherapist. He/she will advise you on how far you should be mobilising and what walking aids are appropriate for you (usually a walking frame initially and then progressing to crutches or sticks).
- It is also important that you carry out some exercises to strengthen the muscles around the damaged hip. These are listed on the following pages. Your physiotherapist may advise you of additional exercises that may also benefit you.
- Because of the position of the wound there is a slight risk of the hip dislocating until the soft tissue around the new hip has healed.
- The advice in this leaflet is designed to help reduce this risk and to help you to get the maximum benefit from your new hip.

To reduce the risks of dislocation follow the precautions below for a period of at least 6 weeks.

1. **Do not bend the operated hip past 90° (a right angle).** Avoid low chairs (your occupational therapist will advise you of your safe sitting height and should check the heights of your chairs at home). Do not raise your knee higher than your hip in sitting, do not lean forwards in sitting (keep your shoulders behind your hips). Do not bend at the waist to pick items up from the floor.
2. **Do not cross your legs.** Always use the dressing aids provided by your occupational therapist.
3. **Do not turn your operated leg inward in a pigeon toe position.** Do not swivel when you turn, always lift your feet. Do not twist your torso while sitting, lying or standing.
4. **Do not roll or lie on the unoperated side.** You may lie on your new hip once it is comfortable to do so, this is usually when the clips are out and the wound is healed.

General advice

Pain - having a joint replacement will relieve the pain from the fracture itself. However, because of the trauma to the soft tissues surrounding the joint during surgery you should expect some pain.

- Taking your medication regularly and following the guidelines in this booklet should help to minimise this.

- On discharge some pain may persist for a further few weeks and you should use this as a guide when increasing your daily activities.

- A moderate ache which settles quickly is acceptable, severe pain which takes hours to settle is not.

- If you experience a sharp pain, stop activity immediately.

- If symptoms persist, contact your physiotherapist for advice.

Swelling - The swelling in the leg may persist for three months or more.

- If the leg is very swollen resting on the bed for an hour or so in the afternoons will help.

- If you wish you may also ice your thigh to help the swelling. You may use crushed ice, a gel pack or a pack of frozen peas which must be wrapped in a damp towel or tea towel before being placed on your thigh.

- Do not keep the ice pack on any longer than 10 minutes. Any longer than this and the body will increase the blood flow to the area in an attempt to warm the tissues up again. This will make the swelling worse. You can have a little as 20 minutes between ice packs.

Infection- Should your wound leak and your dressing need changing before your appointment to have your clips/sutures removed please contact your surgeon to arrange this.

If during the first four weeks after your surgery the wound becomes red, increasingly more painful and/or discharging pus, particularly if you feel unwell with a high temperatures please call the Orthopaedic surgeon.

Mobility/Walking
<u>Standing to use your frame</u>

- Shuffle your bottom to the front of the chair.

- Tuck your feet back underneath you.

- Use the arms of the chair to push up from.

- If it is painful, move the operated leg forwards prior to standing so that more weight is taken on the non-operated leg.

- Once you have your balance reach for your frame.

<u>Sitting down</u>

- Your chair must be high enough so that your knee is lower than your hip.

- Stand close enough to feel the chair against the back of your legs.

- Let go of the frame and reach back to the arms of the chair.

- Slide your operated leg forwards.

- Gently lower yourself in to the chair.

Walking with a frame

- Move the frame first.

- Then step the operated leg forward.

- Push down through the frame and step forward with your non-operated leg.

Points to aim for when walking

- Make sure that both steps are equal in length.

- Try to spend the same amount of time on each leg.

- Always put the heel of each foot to the ground first.

- Gradually increase your walking distance and amount of activity that you do each day.

Getting out of bed
It is not necessary to get out of bed with the operated leg first but you need to be careful to observe the hip precautions shown earlier. In particular, do not let your operated leg cross the midline.

Stairs
Your physiotherapist will practice stairs/steps with you prior to discharge if necessary. You may need to use a stick or crutches on the stairs if you only have one or no rails. You may also need to have extra frame/crutches/sticks to enable you to have something to walk with when you reach the top of the stairs.

Ascending
Hold on to your rail/rails.
Step up with your un-operated leg first, then your operated leg.

- Followed by your stick or crutches.

Descending

- Hold on to your rail/rails.
- Place your crutches or stick down one step.
- Step down with the operated leg first, follow with the un-operated leg.

Getting in/out of the car

- Positioning the car: you should sit in the front passenger seat of the car after your operation as there is more leg room. Make sure the car is parked away from the kerb, so you can be on the same level as the car before you try to get in.
- Push the seat back as far as possible and slightly reclined. Go bottom first into the car and lower yourself slowly to the edge of the seat. Use your arms and lift your bottom further across the seat towards the driver's side. Lift your legs into the car slowly.
- A plastic bag will help you swivel your legs in more slowly, but must be removed before you drive off.
- Reverse this procedure to get out.

Functional activities

- When dressing there are several aids which may be of benefit and these will be supplied by the occupational therapist (OT) i.e. a helping hand, sock aid or long handled shoe horn.
- If your toilet is particularly low a raised toilet seat or toilet frame will be provided by the O.T.
- Use the armrests to get in and out of your chair; the Occupational Therapist will advise you on the best height to sit.
- Follow the advice from your occupational therapist on how to manage in the kitchen and bathroom.

Washing: for the first 6 weeks after your operation you cannot get into a bath as you would break your hip precautions. If your shower is in the bath you will not be able to have a shower for 6 weeks. Having a bath is more likely to take 8-12 weeks as it is the standing up from sitting which is the problem. If you do not have a walk in shower or access to one, you will have to have a stand up strip wash until you can get in the bath. You will require help to wash and dry your feet for the first 6 weeks or you may manage with a combination of a helping hand and/or a long handled brush/sponge.

Dressing:You will not be able to bend down for the first 6 weeks and will therefore need assistance to dress your lower half. The dressing aids recommended by the occupational therapist will make dressing easier. To get dressed: collect your clothes and your three dressing aids and sit somewhere comfortable before you start. The helping hand can be useful for putting on underwear, trousers and skirts until you can bend far enough to do it yourself. It is easier to put your operated leg in first when dressing and last when undressing. The sock aid can be useful for putting on socks until you are flexible enough to do it yourself. The long handled shoe horn can be useful to put your shoes on, and to push your socks, stockings or tights off until you are flexible enough to do it yourself.

In the kitchen:have someone rearrange the contents of your fridge and cupboards so you can reach the more essential items without bending down; stocking the freezer with pre-cooked meals that can be reheated is also useful. A high stool is useful to sit on, for example, when you are preparing vegetables or for eating meals if you are unable to carry it to the dining table.

All heavy worki.e. vacuuming, making beds and cleaning should be done by somebody else.

Driving:In order to drive you need to be nearly pain free, not be dependent on walking aids, have a good range of movement and have sufficient reflexes to manage an emergency stop this is at least six weeks after your operation.

Remember to have a "test drive" and practice an emergency stop with an experienced driver before driving on your own.

It is advisable to contact your motor insurance company before you start driving as this may affect your policy.

Work:Check with the surgeon when you can go back to work.

- If you need a medical certificate for your employer, please ask the nurses before you leave hospital.
- If you have a desk job you will be able to return sooner than if you have a very active job, this will be about 4-8 weeks as compared to 3 months for a physical job.
- Returning to a job that involves some light labour is permitted but those that involve heavy labour are not recommended.

Sports and hobbies:
Recommended activities include walking, swimming, static bike, golf and dancing.

- Sports which involve high impact such as running and jumping should be avoided i.e. jogging, singles tennis, basketball, football.
- Activities such as roller skating, ice skating, horse riding, cycling on the road, downhill skiing maybe recommenced if you have participated in these activities before but they are considered high risk and should not be taken up as a new activity after a total hip replacement.
- Gardening is fine. Long handled tools may be useful when weeding etc and the heavy work should be left for 3 months.

Travelling: It is not advisable to fly within 6 weeks of having a joint replacement due to the increased risk of deep vein thrombosis (blood clot). Long haul flights should be avoided for 3 months.

Exercises

General Precautions:

- TDWB/TTWB for first few weeks (per physician)
- Internal rotation to 0° only (1-12 weeks post-op)
- Adduction to 0° only (1-12 weeks post-op)
- Hip flexion to 90° only (1-12 weeks post-op)

Post -operative
0-4 Weeks
Goals: Safe and independent use of crutches or walker.

- Independent with knowledge and maintenance of hip precautions. Daily performance of home exercise program. All exercises to be repeated 25x, 2-3 x/day. When wound completely healed, begin scar tissue massage.

Exercises:
1. Quad sets- tighten knee muscles of outstretched leg by pushing the back of the knee into the bed, hold 5 seconds.
2. Gluteal sets- squeeze buttocks together, hold 5 seconds.

3. Heel slides- bend knee sliding knee towards buttocks, then slide heel back away from body.

4. Hip abduction & adduction- lay on back, slide straight leg out to side and back in, careful not to cross midline.

5. Short arc quads- put 6 inch towel roll under knee. Straighten lower leg until knee is fully extended and hold for 5 seconds. Then relax and slowly bend knee back to original position.

6. Long arc quads- seated, let legs bend to 90°, straighten lower leg until knee fully extended. Then relax and slowly bend knee down to original position.

4-8 Weeks

Goals: With physician approval, increase weight bearing by 25%/week until 100 % weight bearing. Utilize cane as soon as able and safe. Maintain general hip precautions.

Exercises:

- Stationary bike adjusted to not exceed 90° hip flexion. (When approved by MD)
- Prone hip extension.
- Mini squats.
- Bridges.
- SLR. (Flexion & abduction)
- Hip rotation (No IR, ER to 30°)
- Calf raises.
- Standing hip abduction.
- Standing hip extension.
- Marching.

8-12 Weeks

Goals: Ambulation without device. Ascend and descend stairs in a step over step fashion.

Exercises:

Aquatic Program

- Shallow water walking waist deep.
- SLR in waist deep water (buoyancy assisted and resisted).
- Hip abduction.
- Hip extension.

- Hip flexion to 90°.
- Knee flexion & extension.
- Deep well exercises (bicycle, cross country ski)

General Welness Exercises

Following exercises are to be done immediately after operation to reduce the risk of chest infections and blood clots in the calf.

1. Deep breathing

Breathe in through the nose. Hold for 2-3 second. Breathe out through the mouth. Do 3 or 4 deep breaths.

2. Circulatory exercises - ankle pumps

Point and bend your ankles, a minimum of ten times.
Following exercises should be started the day after your surgery and should be done 10 times each time, four times a day.

1. Static Quads

Lying with legs out straight in front of you, tighten the muscles on the front of your thigh by squashing your knee down into the couch and pulling your toes up towards you. Hold for a count of 6 and relax completely.

2. Gluteal Squeeze

Squeeze your buttock muscles together as tightly as possible for a count of 6, relax completely.

3. Hip Abduction

Lying with your legs out straight in front of you, keeping both legs straight and your toes pointing towards the ceiling throughout, move your operated leg out to the side slowly. Return your leg to the start position, relax completely.

4. Hip Flexion

Lying with your legs out straight in front of you, slide the heel of your operated leg up towards your bottom, allowing your hip and knee to bend. Do not let your hip bend more than a right angle. Slide your heel back down again, relax completely.

5. Long Arc Quadriceps

Sitting on a chair, kick your foot forward and straighten your operated leg slowly, hold for 6 seconds and slowly lower down back. Relax completely.

Following exercises should be started once you are mobile with a frame or crutches and should be done 10 times each time, four times a day.

1. Hip Flexion

In standing, holding a chair for support slowly lift the knee of your operated leg towards your chest. Do not bend your hip more than 90°. Lower your foot back down, relax completely.

2. Hip Extension

In standing, holding a chair for support and keeping your body upright throughout the exercise, slowly move your operated leg as far back as possible. Return to the starting position and relax completely.

3. Hip Abduction

In standing, holding a chair for support and keeping your body upright throughout the exercise, slowly move your operated leg out to the side, keeping your toes pointing forwards. Return to the starting position and relax completely.

4. Hip Hitching

In standing, keeping your body upright throughout the exercise, place your feet together and your legs straight. Shorten one leg to lift the foot. Repeat on other side and relax completely.

2-4 weeks post operatively

1. Half Squats

In standing, holding a chair for support bend both knees. Go as far as you can comfortably then return to the upright position. Repeat 10 times.

2. Heel raises in standing

In standing, holding a chair for support rise up and down on your toes, lifting your heels off the ground. Repeat 10 times.

4-6 weeks post operatively

1. Marching on the spot

In standing, holding a chair on side for support march on the spot for a few minutes.

2. Half Squats

In standing, holding a chair for supports bend both knees as far as comfortable. Repeat 10 times.

3. Hip Abduction in Standing

Stand holding onto the edge of a chair if necessary. Take the operated leg out to the side, hold for a few seconds, relax and return to the middle. Make sure that the toes remain pointing forward and you do not lean to the opposite side. Repeat 10 times.

4. Hip extension in standing

Stand, holding onto the edge of a chair if necessary. Take the operated leg out behind you, taking care not to lean forward at the same time. Hold for a few seconds, relax and repeat 10 times.

After 6 weeks post operatively

- Single leg balance
- Step ups
- Step downs

- Hip extension in prone
- Bridging
- Hip abduction in side lying

CHAPTER NINE

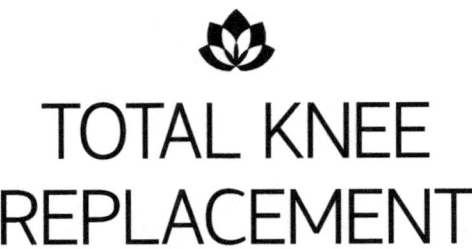

TOTAL KNEE REPLACEMENT

Introduction

Knee replacement/knee arthroplasty, is a surgical procedure to replace the weight-bearing surfaces of the knee joint to relieve pain and disability. It is most commonly performed for osteoarthritis, and also for other knee diseases such as rheumatoid arthritis and psoriatic arthritis.

A total knee replacement is a surgical procedure whereby the diseased knee joint is replaced with artificial material. The knee is a hinge joint that provides motion at the point where the thigh meets the lower leg. The femur abuts the large bone of the lower leg (tibia) at the knee joint.

Risk after TKR

- Risks of total knee replacement include blood clots in the legs that can travel to the lungs (pulmonary embolism). Pulmonary embolism can cause shortness of breath, chest pain, and even shock.
- Other risks include urinary tract infection, nausea and vomiting (usually related to pain medication), chronic knee pain and stiffness, bleeding into the knee joint, nerve damage, blood vessel injury, and infection of the knee which can require reoperation. Furthermore, the risks of anaesthesia include potential heart, lung, kidney, and liver damage.

Physiotherapy Guidelines

This is a guideline for you physiotherapist to help you progress through rehabilitation over the course of 12 weeks following your knee operation. A physiotherapist who is experienced in knee rehabilitation should be consulted throughout the programme to supervise and where necessary individually modify your programme.

Aims of Rehabilitation

To restore range of motion and strength of the knee. The final goal is to minimize knee pain and improve your knee function to improve your quality of life.

Type of Replacement Performed

Total Knee Replacement
Unicompartmental Knee Replacement

- Medial
- Lateral
- Patello-femoral

Post Operative Programme
1-14 Days
Manual Physiotherapy

- Intermittent cryotherapy to minimize joint swelling over first 4-5 days.
- Cryotherapy after exercises. Heat packs may be used on the knee and thigh prior to exercises.
- Circumferential compression dressing (Tubigrip) from ankle to thigh.
- Elevate the affected limb to minimize swelling.
- Ankle exercises for Deep Vein Thrombosis prophylaxis.
- Deep breathing exercises for basal atelectasis.

Range of Motion / Strengthening Exercises

– Quadriceps sets and Gluteal sets.
– Straight leg raises in supine.
– Knee extensions in supine over a roll.
– Knee extensions from seated posture
– Passive knee straightening with a heel roll in supine.
– Heel slides in seated and supine.

Functional Exercises

– Transfer lying to standing, and seated to standing.
– Gait training with crutches, including stairs.
– Into and out of a car.
– Weight bear as tolerated.

3-6 weeks
Manual Physiotherapy

– Cryotherapy after exercises, heat packs may be used on the knee and thigh prior to exercises.
– Circumferential compression dressing (Tubigrip) from ankle to thigh.
– Ankle exercises for DVT prophylaxis.
– Patellar mobilization exercises.
– Quads and hamstrings deep tissue massage.

Range of Motion / Strengthening Exercises
– Isometric quads, hamstrings, gluteals, adductors.
– Core stabilizing exercises.
– Active and assisted range of motion exercises.
– Supported standing heel raises, calf stretches, mini squats, hamstring curls.
– Hydrotherapy after week 3.

Functional Activities
– Gait – normalize gait between crutches, progressing to a single point stick.
– Weight bearing as tolerated.
– Increase endurance with longer walks and stairs.

Patients should be walking without aids and achieving flexion >90° by 6 weeks post-operation

7-12 weeks

Manual Physiotherapy
– Patellar mobilization exercises.
– Quads and hamstrings deep tissue massage.
– Wound massage with Bio-oil or Vitamin E cream.

Range of Motion / Strengthening Exercises
– Core stabilization exercises.
– Squats and single leg stance mini-squats.
– Resistance exercises for quadriceps, hamstrings, gluteals and adductors.
– Active and assisted ROM exercises.

Functional Exercises
– Start driving using the affected leg.
– Gait supervision without walking aids.
– Lateral stepping.
– Heel-toe walking.
– Exercise bike (can start earlier if good balance).

13+ weeks

Training for good Life

Once the patient has achieved full extension and flexion >110°, normalized and unaided gait, and good muscle balance – institute an ongoing programme of regular exercise tailored to the patient.

This may include:
- Regular walking
- Exercise bike
- Hydrotherapy
- Gentle gym workouts
- Return to sport (golf, doubles tennis, lawn bowls, etc)

Encourage the patient to continue their exercise program *indefinitely*, to optimize the outcome from their surgery.

CHAPTER TEN

SPECIAL TESTS OF LOWER EXTREMITY

Hip and pelvis special tests

1. **Ely's Test**

    Test for: Rectus Femoris Contracture
    Procedure: patient in prone lying. Flex the patient's affected side knee. Try to bring the heel to glutes. Prevent abduction of testing or affected leg.
    Positive sign: the affected side pelvis flexes as therapist try to get the heel touch to affected side glutes.

2. **Faber Test**

    Test for: Hip pathology and Psoas muscle spasm or shortness.
    Procedure: patient in supine lying and both the legs extended. Place patient's foot of the affected side on the sound or other knee.
    Positive sign: the affected side hip stays above level of the sound knee and pain may be present.

3. **Gaenslen's Test**

    Test for: Hip or Sacroiliac Joint Dysfunction
    Procedure: patient is side lying on the unaffected side. Patient flexes the hip and knee of the unaffected leg towards his chest. Therapist stands behind the patient, stabilizes patient's pelvis with one hand. Therapist then hyper-extends the patient's affected leg at the hip.
    Positive Sign: Pain present in the hip and SI joint area.

4. **Ober's Test**

   Test for: The length of the Iliotibial band and Tensor Fascia Lata
   Procedure: Patient is side lying close to the edge of the table on the unaffected leg. Therapist stands behind the Patient. Flex hip and knee of the unaffected leg that is at the bottom. Stabilize the Patient's pelvis with one hand. With the other hand grasping the medial aspect of the patient's affected knee, passively hyper-abduct and extend theaffected femur at the hip. Allow the affected leg to lower without rotating
   Positive Sign: the affected leg stays abducted and does not lower.

5. **Gillet's Test**

   Test for: Mobility of the Sacroiliac joint
   Procedure: Patient is standing, may hold on to something for stability. Therapist is behind the patient. Therapist palpates the PSIS of the patient's affected side with their thumb. Therapist places their other thumb on the S2 process of the patient's sacrum. Patient flexes the hip and knee of the affected side, raising their knee as high as they can, while standing on the unaffected side.
   Positive Sign: SI joint hypomobility if the thumb on the affected side moves superiorly instead of inferiorly as the knee lifts.

6. **Straight Leg Raise**

   Test for: determine the cause of low back pain
   Procedure: Patient is supine. Place their affected leg in adduction and internal rotation. Raise the affected leg by grasping it around the heel and flexing the hip (their affected knee should be extended). Flex the hip until the patient feels pain (usually around 70-80 degrees of flexion). Slowly lower the leg until no pain is felt by the patient. Dorsi flex the patient's affected foot (this stretches their sciatic nerve).
   Positive Signs:

   - Hamstring Tightness – pain in the back of their thigh and knee during hip flexion.
   - Lumbar or SI Joint Dysfunction – pain in the low back after 70 degrees of hip flexion only (no foot dorsi flexion).

- Sciatic Nerve Involvement – pain down the leg during passive dorsi flexion.
- Space Occupying Lesion or Disc Herniation – pain down their opposite leg (the one that is not raised).

7. **Thomas Test**

    Test for: Hip flexor muscle contracture or shortness
    Procedure: Patient is supine, with lower gluteal folds at the end of the table and their hips and knees flexed. Patient may hold thelegs in flexion with their hands.Therapist makes sure that the patient's lower back is not so high off the table.Patient keeps the unaffected leg flexed, and slowly lowers the affected leg and lets it extend as far as it can
    Positive Sign:

- Short Quadriceps: the affected knee stays extended
- Short Psoas muscles: the hips remains flexed
- Short TFL/ ITB: Abducted hip

8. **Trendelenburg's Sign**

    Test for: the strength of the Gluteus Medius Muscle
    Procedure: Patient is standing. Therapist stands behind patient, paying attention to the patient's PSIS and iliac spines. Patient stands on the affected leg.
    Positive Sign: gluteus medius is weak if the pelvis on the affected side pops out or drops.

    Knee Tests

1. **True Tibia and Femur Length Test**

    Test for: The tibia and femur lengths
    Procedure: Patient is prone. Patient's knees and hips flexed, with the plantar surfaces of their feet on the table. Their medial malleoli even and knees togetherto compare the lengths of:

- Tibia: Therapist stands at the foot of the table to compare the heights of the patient's tibial plateaus to look for the shorter tibia.
- Femur: Then therapist stands at the side of the table to compare the positions of the patellas looking for the shorter femur.

2. **Noble's Test**

   Test for: The presence of iliotibial band (ITB) friction syndrome
   Procedure: Patient is supine, with both their affected side's knee and hip flexed to 90° degrees. Therapist compresses the iliotibial band (ITB) 2 centimetres proximal to the lateral femoral condyle. Instruct the patient to extend the knee and hip slowly while therapist maintains compression of the ITB proximal to the lateral femoral condyle.
   Positive Sign: Pain over the lateral femoral condyle at about 30° degrees of knee extension.

3. **Gravity Drawer Test/ Posterior Sign**

   Test for: To assess the integrity of the posterior cruciate ligament.
   Procedure: Patient is supine, their hips flexed to 45 degrees and their knees flexed to 90 degrees and their feet are flat on the table. Observe the profile of both knees from the side of the table
   Positive Sign: The affected tibia sags posteriorly compared to the unaffected knee. (In given position, the tibia drops posteriorly on thefemur if the posterior cruciate ligament's integrity is compromised).

4. **Waldron's Test**

   Test for: The Presence of patellofemoral syndrome.
   Procedure: Patient is standing. Therapist palpates the patella while the patient performs knee bends.
   Positive Sign: Presence of pain, crepitus, poor patellar tracking.

5. **Major Effusion Test/Ballottable Patella**

   Test for: Usually performed after an injury to assess for a major increase in the synovial fluid or blood within the knee joint capsule.

Procedure: Patient is supine, the affected knee is extended as much as possible (with effusion, patient may not be able to extendtheir knee fully). Therapist gently extends the knee further, then compresses the patella down on to the condyles then release.

Positive Sign: Patella clicks onto the femur and then rebounds to the floating position. This could be caused by torn cruciateligaments, meniscal tearing, or fracture and is considered a Medical Emergency. (Joint effusion within two hours ofinjury might be caused by blood in the joint, and joint effusion with synovial fluid usually develops 8 hours after injury)

6. **Minor Effusion Test/Brush Test**

Test for: To assess for lesser amounts of synovial fluid within the knee joint right after an injury. This is usually done after the Major Effusion Test comes up negative.

Procedure: Patient is supine; their affected knee is extended as much as they canTherapist slowly sweeps the effusion from the superior lateral aspect of the knee and suprapatellar pouch

Positive Sign: A bulge inferior to the patella appears within two seconds, the positive test will indicate from 4-8 millimeters of extrasynovial fluid within the joint. This could be caused by cruciate or meniscal damage and is considered a MedicalEmergency.

7. **Q-Angle**

The Q angle is the angle between the quadriceps tendon and the patellar tendon. The Q-angle is formed from a line drawn from the ASIS to the centre of the kneecap, and from the centre of the kneecap to the tibial tubercle. To find the Q-angle, measure that angle, and subtract from 180 degrees.

Procedure: Patient is standing, with the knee in extension and femur neutral: (no internal or external rotation) and patient's feet in a neutral position (no pronation or supination).

Normal Q Angle Test Result:

A normal Q angle with the knee extended and the quadriceps muscle relaxed is 18° degrees for women and 13° degrees for men.

- A Q angle that is less than normal allows the patella to track medially between femoral condyles, placing extra stress on the medial articulating facets of the patella which leads to Chondromalacia Patellae.
- A Q angle that is greater than normal allows the patella to track laterally, stressing the lateral facet which is associated with patellar tracking dysfunction, chondromalacia patellae and patellar subluxation.

8. **Valgus Stress Test of the Knee**

Test for: The integrity of the structures that prevent Valgus deformity of the knee (Joint capsule, medial collateral ligament, cruciate ligaments).

Procedure: Patient is supine. Place the affected leg in extension and slight external rotation.

Stabilize with one hand on the medial malleolus and with the other hand stabilize the lateral aspect of the knee. Apply a medially directed stress on the lateral knee. Flex his knee to 30 degrees and apply the same pressure on the lateral side to isolate the medial collateral ligament.

Positive Sign: Presence of pain and hypermobility at the medial aspect of the knee.

9. **Varus Stress Test of the Knee**

Test for: The integrity of the structures that prevent lateral instability at the knee (lateral collateral ligament, joint capsule, cruciate ligaments).

Procedure: Patient is supine with the affected knee in full extension. Therapist stabilizes the affected leg in slight external rotation with one hand on the lateral malleolus. Therapist places their other hand on the medial aspect of the knee. Therapist applies a laterally directed/varus stress on the medial knee. Flex their knee to 30 degrees and apply the same pressure on the lateral side to isolate the lateral collateral ligament.

Positive Sign: Presence of pain and hypermobility at the lateral aspect of the knee.

10. **Lachman's Test**

Test for: The integrity of the Anterior Cruciate Ligament (ACL). The Lachman's test is considered to be the most accurate test for ACL integrity.

Procedure: Patient is supine. Patient's affected knee is flexed 30°. Therapist stabilizes distal femur with one hand while grasping patient's proximal tibia with the other hand. Therapist applies an anteriorly directed stress the tibia.

Positive Sign: Pain or excessive anterior motion of the tibia, and disappearance of the infrapatellar tendon slope.

11. **Patellar Apprehension Test**

    Test for: To test whether the patella is likely to dislocate laterally.
    Procedure: Patient is supine with their affected knee extended. Therapist uses a slow and moderate pressure against the medial aspect of the patella moving it in a lateral direction. Therapist observes patient's reaction.
    Positive Sign: Patient expresses apprehension and/ or might try to move their affected knee away from the pressure.

12. **McMurray's Test**

    Test for: Injury to the Menisci.
    Procedure: Patient is supine, their affected hip and knee are flexed. Therapist cups one hand over the patient's knee (palm over the patella and fingers/thumb over the joint line). Therapist grasps patient's heel with the other hand. Therapist slowly extends the patient's knee, while applying different stresses to check both menisci:

    - external rotation of the tibia and valgus stress on the knee to assess medial meniscus
    - internal rotation of the tibia and varus stress on the knee to assess lateral meniscus

    Positive Sign: Click or catch in the extension of the knee.

13. **Apley's Compression Test (Knee)**

    Test for: Meniscal Injury
    Procedure: Patient is prone. Patient then flexes affected knee to 90°. Therapist's one hand grasps patient's heel and ankle while the other hand

stabilizes the leg. Therapist compresses the flexed knee joint and the menisci by pushing the patient's foot and tibia down into thetable, followed by internal and external rotation of the tibia.

Positive Sign: Pain on the medial aspect indicates medial meniscus injury.

Pain on the lateral aspect indicates lateral meniscus injury.

14. Apley's Distraction Test

Test for: The Integrity of the Collateral Knee Ligaments.

Procedure: Patient is prone, with their affected knee flexed to 90°. Therapist places their own knee on patient's posterior thigh to stabilize. Therapist grasps patient's leg proximal to the ankle. Therapist applies traction to the tibia towards the ceiling to distract the knee joint. Then apply internal andexternal rotation of the tibia while maintaining traction.

Positive Sign:

- Pain on the medial side indicates medial collateral ligament injury.
- Pain on the lateral side indicates lateral collateral ligament injury.

15. Clarke's Patellofemoral Grind Test

Test for: Patellofemoral Syndrome.

Procedure: Patient is supine with their knees extended. Therapist compresses the patella posteriorly onto the femoral condyles and then, moderately move the patella distally. Therapist instructs patient to contract the quadriceps muscles to pull patella proximally.

Positive Sign: Pain, crepitus, apprehension of the patient as the irritated surfaces of the patella rub over the femur.

16. McConnell's Test

Test for: Patellofemoral Tracking problems.
Procedure:
Method I: Patient is seated with legs hanging over the end of the table. Therapist sits in front of the patient. Therapist instructs patient to externally rotate the femur of the affected leg while performing active resisted isometriccontractions of the quadriceps muscles at 0, 30, 60, 90 and

120 degrees of flexion. Therapist notes the painful degrees/ ranges.

Method II: Therapist passively brings the patient's knee to full extension, resting the heel on something so the patient relaxes thequadriceps musclesthen, Therapist glides the affected patella medially and hold the patella it in that position. Therapist instructs patient to perform isometric contractions at the knee ranges that were painful before.

Method III: Therapist passively brings the patient's knee to full extension, resting the heel on something so the patient relaxes thequadriceps musclesthen, Therapist glides the affected patella laterally and hold the patella it in that position. Therapist instructs patient to perform isometric contractions at the knee ranges that were painful before.

Positive Test:

- Pain decreases significantly after holding patella medially indicates patellofemoral lateral tracking problems and/or;
- Pain decreases significantly after holding patella laterally indicates patellofemoral medial tracking problems.

Ankle & Foot Special Tests:

1. **Anterior Drawer Test (Ankle)**

Test for: Anterior Talofibular Ligament injury and/ or ligamentous instability.

Procedure: Patient is supine with foot relaxed. Therapist stabilizes tibia and fibula with one hand. With the Patient's foot plantar flexed to 20 degrees, the therapist holds the patient's calcaneus with other hand thendistracts the calcaneus from the tibia and fibula (by slowly pulling the calcanues inferiorly). Therapist places an anteriorly directed pressure on the calcaneus and talus, applying overpressure at the end of thepassive range (stressing the Anterior Talofibular ligament).

Positive Sign: Ligamentous laxity or rupture with presence of sulcus and pain, and/ or excessive anterior translation of the talus, sometimes accompanied by audible clunking.

2. **Deltoid Ligamentous Stress Test**

Test for: To assess the deltoid ligament using 3 separate passive movements.

Procedure: Patient is seated with their leg flexed at the knee and hanging over a table. Therapist stabilizes the anterior surface of the tibia and fibula proximal to the ankle (with one hand) and

- Test Anterior Fibers of the Deltoid Ligament:

Therapist uses his other hand to grap the dorsal surface of the foot, combining eversion and plantarflexion of the foot and applying overpressure.

- Test Middle Fibers of the Deltoid Ligament:

Therapist repositions his hand so the calcaneus is grasped (still stabilizing the anterior surface of the tibia and fibula proximal to the ankle with their other hand). Hind foot is taken into eversion with overpressure.

- Test Posterior Fibers of the Deltoid Ligament:

Therapist repositions his hand so the calcaneus is grasped (still stabilizing the anterior surface of the tibia and fibula proximal to the ankle with their other hand). Therapist combines eversion and dorsiflexion of the foot with overpressure.

Note: to perform a general assessment of the deltoid ligament, evert the hind foot only.

Positive Sign: Pain and Hypermobility local to the ligament. Muscle spasm end feel may be present with a subacute injury.

3. **Functional or Structural Pes Planus (Flat foot) Test**

Test for: To determine whether a pes planus is functional or structural.

Procedure: Therapist observes (and compares) the orientation of the patient's medial longitudinal arch while doing each of thefollowing:

- Patient stands straight with both heels and toes on the ground.
- Patient stands with just the toes on the ground.
- Patient sits on the table.

Positive Sign:
Functional Pes Planus present if medial longitudinal arch is restored when the patient is either standing on the toes or seated which is due to muscle or ligament weakness.

Structural Pes Planus present if medial longitudinal arch remains flat when the patient is standing on toes and when seated.

4. Homan's Sign

Test for: The presence of Deep Vein Thrompophlebitis / Deep Vein Thrombosis.

Procedure: patient supine with the knee extended. Patient's foot is passively dorsi flexed.

Positive Signs: Pain deep in the calf during dorsi flexionand also tenderness elicited on palpation of the calf, pallor and swelling in leg, and loss of dorsalis pedis artery pulse.

5. Morton's Neuroma Test

Test for: The presence of Morton's Neuroma.

Morton's Neuroma (is a benign neuroma of an intermetatarsal plantar nerve, most commonly of the second and third intermetatarsal spaces (between 3rd-4th metatarsal heads). This problem is characterised by pain and/or numbness, sometimes relieved by removing footwear.

Procedure: Patient is seated. Compress the foot by applying pressure to the medial and lateral aspects of the foot at the metatarsophalangel joints.

Positive Sign: Sharp pain at the location of the neuroma. Pain is worsend by activity.

6. Posterior Drawer Test (Ankle)

Test for: Posterior Talofibular ligament injury and/or ligamentous instability.

Procedure: Patient is supine with foot relaxed. Therapist stabilizes tibia and fibula with one hand. With the patient's foot plantar flexed to 20 degrees, the Therapist holds the patient's calcaneus with other hand then distracts the calcaneus from the tibia and fibula (by slowly pulling the calcanues inferiorly). Therapist places an posteriorly directed pressure on the calcaneus and talus, applying overpressure at the end of the passive range.

Positive Sign: Ligamentous laxity or rupture with presence of sulcus and pain, and/ or

excessive posterior translation of the talus.

7. **Thompson's Test (Achilles Tendon rupture)**

Test for: 3rd degree strain or rupture of the Achilles tendon
Procedure: Patient is prone lying, feet over the edge of the table, legs relaxed. Squeeze the affected gastrocnemius and soleus muscles.
Positive Sign: Absence of plantarflexion when the muscles are squeezed.

8. **Tinel's Sign (Ankle)**

Test for: Anterior or Posterior Tibial Nerve entrapment or dysfunction.
Procedure: Anterior tibial branch of deep peroneal nerve is tapped in front of the ankle.
The Posterior tibial nerve tapped as it passes behind the medial malleolus.
Positive Sign: Tingling or Paresthesia felt distally.

References

1. Frymoyer, John W. "Back pain and sciatica." *New England Journal of Medicine* 318.5 (1988): 291-300.
2. Heliövaara, M. A. R. K. K. U., et al. "Determinants of sciatica and low-back pain." *Spine* 16.6 (1991): 608-614.
3. Koes, Bart W., M. W. Van Tulder, and W. C. Peul. "Diagnosis and treatment of sciatica." *Bmj* 334.7607 (2007): 1313-1317.
4. Parziale, J. R., T. H. Hudgins, and L. M. Fishman. "The piriformis syndrome." *American journal of orthopedics (Belle Mead, NJ)* 25.12 (1996): 819-823.
5. Fishman, Loren M., and Patricia A. Zybert. "Electrophysiologic evidence of piriformis syndrome." *Archives of physical medicine and rehabilitation* 73.4 (1992): 359-364.
6. Benson, Eric R., and Steven F. Schutzer. "Posttraumatic piriformis syndrome: diagnosis and results of operative treatment." *JBJS* 81.7 (1999): 941.
7. Keskula, Douglas R., and Michael Tamburello. "Conservative management of piriformis syndrome." *Journal of athletic training* 27.2 (1992): 102.
8. Cramp, Fiona, et al. "Non-surgical management of piriformis syndrome: a systematic review." *Physical therapy reviews* 12.1 (2007): 66-72.
9. Cass, Shane P. "Piriformis syndrome: a cause of nondiscogenic sciatica." *Current sports medicine reports* 14.1 (2015): 41-44.
10. Larsson, Maria EH, Ingela Käll, and Katarina Nilsson-Helander. "Treatment of patellar tendinopathy—a systematic review of randomized controlled trials." *Knee surgery, sports traumatology, arthroscopy* 20.8 (2012): 1632-1646.
11. Van der Worp, Henk, et al. "Risk factors for patellar tendinopathy: a systematic review of the literature." *Br J Sports Med* 45.5 (2011): 446-452.
12. Liddle, Alexander D., and E. Carlos Rodríguez-Merchán. "Platelet-rich plasma in the treatment of patellar tendinopathy: a systematic review." *The American journal of sports medicine* 43.10 (2015): 2583-2590.

13. Rudavsky, Aliza, and Jill Cook. "Physiotherapy management of patellar tendinopathy (jumper's knee)." *Journal of physiotherapy* 60.3 (2014): 122-129.
14. Cook, Jill L., Karim M. Khan, and Craig R. Purdam. "Conservative treatment of patellar tendinopathy." *Physical Therapy in Sport* 2.2 (2001): 54-65.
15. Lipscomb, A. Brant, E. Dewey Thomas, and Robert K. Johnston. "Treatment of myositis ossificans traumatica in athletes." *The American journal of sports medicine* 4.3 (1976): 111-120.
16. Wieder, Deborah L. "Treatment of traumatic myositis ossificans with acetic acid iontophoresis." *Physical therapy* 72.2 (1992): 133-137.
17. GESCHICKTER, CHARLES F., and I. H. Maseritz. "Myositis ossificans." *JBJS* 20.3 (1938): 661-674.
18. Parikh, J., H. Hyare, and A. Saifuddin. "The imaging features of post-traumatic myositis ossificans, with emphasis on MRI." *Clinical radiology* 57.12 (2002): 1058-1066.
19. Della Croce, Ugo, Aurelio Cappozzo, and D. Casey Kerrigan. "Pelvis and lower limb anatomical landmark calibration precision and its propagation to bone geometry and joint angles." *Medical & biological engineering & computing* 37.2 (1999): 155-161.
20. Sailhan, Frédéric, Louis Jacob, and Moussa Hamadouche. "Differences in limb alignment and femoral mechanical-anatomical angles using two dimension versus three dimension radiographic imaging." *International orthopaedics* 41.10 (2017): 2009-2016.
21. Brennan, A., K. Deluzio, and Q. Li. "Assessment of anatomical frame variation effect on joint angles: A linear perturbation approach." *Journal of biomechanics* 44.16 (2011): 2838-2842.
22. Nordqvist, Anders, and Claes J. Petersson. "Shoulder injuries common in alcoholics: An analysis of 413 injuries." *Acta Orthopaedica Scandinavica* 67.4 (1996): 364-366.
23. Maffulli, Nicola, and Adam DG Baxter-Jones. "Common skeletal injuries in young athletes." *Sports Medicine* 19.2 (1995): 137-149.
24. Peskun, Christopher J., et al. "Diagnosis and management of knee dislocations." *The Physician and sportsmedicine* 38.4 (2010): 101-111.
25. Levine, Robert S. "A review of the long-term effects of selected lower limb injuries." *SAE transactions* (1986): 370-385.
26. Yamamoto, Yasuhiro, et al. "Arthroscopic surgery to treat intra-articular type snapping hip." *Arthroscopy: The Journal of Arthroscopic & Related*

Surgery 21.9 (2005): 1120-1125.
27. Torisu, T., S. Yosida, and M. Takasita. "Painful snapping in rheumatoid knees." *International orthopaedics* 21.6 (1998): 361-363.
28. Wunderbaldinger, P., et al. "Efficient radiological assessment of the internal snapping hip syndrome." *European radiology* 11.9 (2001): 1743-1747.
29. Steinert, Andre F., et al. "Snapping elbow caused by hypertrophic synovial plica in the radiohumeral joint: a report of three cases and review of literature." *Archives of orthopaedic and trauma surgery* 130.3 (2010): 347-351.
30. Bae, Dae Kyung, and Oh Soo Kwon. "Snapping knee caused by the gracilis and semitendinosus tendon. A case report." *Bulletin (Hospital for Joint Diseases (New York, NY))* 56.3 (1997): 177-179.
31. Aoki, Mitsuhiro, Kenji Okamura, and Toshihiko Yamashita. "Snapping annular ligament of the elbow joint in the throwing arms of young brothers." *Arthroscopy: The Journal of Arthroscopic & Related Surgery* 19.8 (2003): e89-e92.
32. Wohlrab, D., A. Hagel, and W. Hein. "Advantages of minimal invasive total hip replacement in the early phase of rehabilitation." *Zeitschrift fur Orthopadie und ihre Grenzgebiete* 142.6 (2004): 685-690.
33. Coulter, Corinne L., et al. "Physiotherapist-directed rehabilitation exercises in the outpatient or home setting improve strength, gait speed and cadence after elective total hip replacement: a systematic review." *Journal of physiotherapy* 59.4 (2013): 219-226.
34. Iyengar, Karthikeyan P., et al. "Targeted early rehabilitation at home after total hip and knee joint replacement: does it work?." *Disability and rehabilitation* 29.6 (2007): 495-502.
35. Herbold, Janet A., Kristen Bonistall, and Mary Beth Walsh. "Rehabilitation following total knee replacement, total hip replacement, and hip fracture: a case-controlled comparison." *Journal of geriatric physical therapy* 34.4 (2011): 155-160.
36. Okoro, Tosan, et al. "An appraisal of rehabilitation regimes used for improving functional outcome after total hip replacement surgery." *Sports Medicine, Arthroscopy, Rehabilitation, Therapy & Technology* 4.1 (2012): 5.
37. Heaton, J. A. N. E. T., et al. "Rehabilitation and total hip replacement: patients' perspectives on provision." *International journal of rehabilitation research. Internationale Zeitschrift fur Rehabilitationsforschung. Revue*

REFERENCES

internationale de recherches de readaptation 23.4 (2000): 253-259.
38. Peersman, G., et al. "Infection in total knee replacement: a retrospective review of 6489 total knee replacements." *Clinical Orthopaedics and Related Research®* 392 (2001): 15-23.
39. Bradbury, Neil, et al. "Participation in sports after total knee replacement." *The American journal of sports medicine* 26.4 (1998): 530-535.
40. Ibrahim, M. S., et al. "An evidence-based review of enhanced recovery interventions in knee replacement surgery." *The Annals of The Royal College of Surgeons of England* 95.6 (2013): 386-389.
41. Artz, Neil, et al. "Effectiveness of physiotherapy exercise following total knee replacement: systematic review and meta-analysis." *BMC musculoskeletal disorders* 16.1 (2015): 15.
42. Mitchell, Caroline, et al. "Costs and effectiveness of pre-and post-operative home physiotherapy for total knee replacement: randomized controlled trial." *Journal of evaluation in clinical practice* 11.3 (2005): 283-292.
43. Skou, Søren T., et al. "A randomized, controlled trial of total knee replacement." *New England Journal of Medicine* 373.17 (2015): 1597-1606.
44. Harmer, Alison R., et al. "Land-based versus water-based rehabilitation following total knee replacement: A randomized, single-blind trial." *Arthritis Care & Research* 61.2 (2009): 184-191.
45. Rahmann, Ann E., Sandra G. Brauer, and Jennifer C. Nitz. "A specific inpatient aquatic physiotherapy program improves strength after total hip or knee replacement surgery: a randomized controlled trial." *Archives of physical medicine and rehabilitation* 90.5 (2009): 745-755.
46. Magee, David J. *Orthopedic physical assessment*. Elsevier Health Sciences, 2013.
47. Scopp, Jason M., and Claude T. Moorman. "The assessment of athletic hip injury." *Clinics in sports medicine* 20.4 (2001): 647-660.
48. Hamblen, David L., and Hamish Simpson. *Adams's Outline of Orthopaedics E-Book*. Elsevier Health Sciences, 2009.
49. Solomon, Louis, David Warwick, and Selvadurai Nayagam, eds. *Apley's system of orthopaedics and fractures*. CRC press, 2010.

www.ingramcontent.com/pod-product-compliance
Lightning Source LLC
Chambersburg PA
CBHW070813220526
45466CB00002B/653